LYMPHATIC PROBLEMS RESOLVED

Therapies For Detoxification And Immune Support

A Comprehensive Guide To Relief And Completely Treat Your Body System For A Healthy Life

DR. BRIDGET PROMISE

Introduction

The human body is a complex network of interrelated systems that work together to keep us healthy and balanced. The lymphatic system is a vital system that sometimes goes unseen but plays an important role in immune function and general health.

This complex network of veins, nodes, and organs is in charge of maintaining fluid balance, filtering pollutants, and assisting the body's fight against infection. Understanding the lymphatic system, detecting possible problems, and comprehending the value of cleansing are all critical components of sustaining good health.

Understanding The Lymphatic System

The lymphatic system is a complicated network that runs parallel to the circulatory system, working together to maintain the body in balance.

This system, which includes lymph nodes, arteries, tonsils, spleen, and thymus, is responsible for the circulation and filtration of lymph, a colorless fluid containing white blood cells, proteins, and waste materials. Unlike the circulatory system, the lymphatic system lacks a pump and instead relies on muscle contractions, breathing, and physical activity to transfer lymph.

fluid nodes serve as checkpoints throughout the body by filtering fluid and capturing foreign particles including bacteria, viruses, and aberrant cells.

The spleen, which is positioned on the left side of the abdomen, functions as a blood filter by eliminating damaged blood cells and functioning as a storage for immune cells. The thymus, located beneath the breastbone, is critical in the development of T lymphocytes, a kind of white blood cell required for immunological responses.

The lymphatic system's major role is to convey lymph, which contains infection-fighting cells and nutrients, while also eliminating waste and toxins. This sophisticated network maintains a delicate balance by boosting immune responses and protecting the body from dangerous intruders.

Signs And Symptoms Of Lymphatic Conditions

While the lymphatic system is intended to work properly, a variety of circumstances may contribute to its malfunction, resulting in a variety of indications and symptoms. Recognizing these markers is critical for treating any problems and preserving general health.

Swelling or edema is a typical symptom of lymphatic issues. When the lymphatic system fails to drain fluid properly, fluid may accumulate in tissues, producing edema, especially in the extremities. This disorder, called lymphedema, may result from surgery, injury, or an underlying medical condition that impairs lymphatic function.

Chronic weariness is another sign that might suggest lymphatic problems. The lymphatic system removes waste and poisons from the body. If this process is disrupted, the accumulation of pollutants may lead to sensations of exhaustion and sluggishness.

Recurrent infections or a weaker immune system might potentially be signs of lymphatic issues.

Skin problems such as dryness, itching, or redness may indicate lymphatic insufficiency. The skin is an important organ for detoxification, and when the lymphatic system fails to discharge waste, it may cause a variety of skin disorders.

Understanding these signs and symptoms enables people to seek medical care as soon as possible, allowing for early detection and treatment of any lymphatic disorders.

CHAPTER TWO

Importance Of Detoxification

Detoxification is a procedure that removes or neutralizes toxic chemicals from the body. While numerous organs aid in detoxification, the lymphatic system is critical in the elimination of waste and toxins, protecting the body's interior environment.

The lymphatic system's purpose in detoxification is to filter and move lymph, which transports waste products and toxins away from cells and tissues. Lymph nodes serve as essential gatekeepers, capturing and neutralizing dangerous chemicals before they may spread throughout the body. Additionally, the spleen and thymus aid in detoxification by filtering and cleaning the blood.

Maintaining a healthy and efficient lymphatic system is critical for successful detoxification. Adequate hydration is essential for lymphatic function because water is required to carry nutrients and remove waste via the lymphatic vessels. A proper diet is also important since it provides the body with the nutrients it needs for proper lymphatic function.

Regular physical exercise naturally stimulates the lymphatic system. Exercise stimulates muscular contractions, which help in the circulation of lymph throughout the body. Activities like rebounding, yoga, and brisk walking may help improve lymphatic circulation.

Deep breathing and massage are two examples of relaxation methods that might help in detoxification. Stress management is critical because prolonged stress may impede lymphatic function and the body's capacity to remove toxins.

Various holistic treatments, such as dry brushing and hydrotherapy, are becoming popular due to their ability to activate the lymphatic system and promote cleansing. Dry brushing is the process of gently massaging the skin with a brush with soft bristles, which promotes lymphatic movement and exfoliation. Hydrotherapy, which involves contrast showers or hot and cold water treatments, may stimulate the circulatory and lymphatic systems.

To summarize, knowing the complexities of the lymphatic system, detecting warning signals of possible problems, and accepting the significance of detoxification are all essential components of holistic health. Individuals may improve their general health by raising knowledge and implementing actions that promote lymphatic function and cleansing.

The lymphatic system, a fundamental component of the body's immune system, is essential for general health and wellness. This system, which consists of a network of lymph nodes, veins, and organs, filters and drains lymph, a fluid containing white blood cells, throughout the body.

When the lymphatic system works properly, it boosts immune function and aids in the elimination of pollutants. However, sedentary lifestyles, poor food choices, and stress may all cause slow lymphatic drainage, possibly leading to a variety of health disorders.

Natural Treatments For Lymphatic Support

Several natural therapies are thought to improve lymphatic support, detoxification, and immune system function. One such therapy is dry brushing, which involves gently exfoliating the skin with a natural bristle brush.

This approach is supposed to stimulate the lymphatic system by increasing the flow of lymph and improving waste elimination. Dry brushing, when done consistently, may help to improve circulation and minimize lymphatic congestion.

Herbal Teas Are Another Popular natural lymphatic support therapy. Certain plants, including echinacea, cleavers, and red clover, are thought to improve lymphatic drainage and boost the immune system. These teas may be a relaxing and delightful approach to including lymphatic health practices in your everyday routine.

Essential oils, especially those with detoxifying characteristics, are often utilized in aromatherapy to enhance lymphatic function. Oils such as grapefruit, lemon, and cypress are thought to increase lymphatic circulation when applied topically or diffused. Additionally, adding these essential oils to a soothing bath might improve the entire therapeutic experience.

CHAPTER THREE

Dietary strategies for lymphatic detoxification

A nutrient-dense, well-balanced diet is essential for maintaining proper lymphatic function. Certain meals are thought to enhance the body's natural detoxification processes and promote lymphatic health.

Hydration is essential; drinking enough water helps eliminate toxins from the body and promotes lymph movement. Lemon is known to stimulate the lymphatic system, so adding it to water may give it an additional kick.

Other dietary strategies for lymphatic detoxification include including antioxidant-rich foods. Berries, leafy greens, and citrus fruits are antioxidant-rich foods that may help neutralize free radicals and minimize oxidative stress on the lymphatic system. Furthermore, eating a fiber-rich diet promotes good digestion by reducing the buildup of waste materials that might stress the lymphatic system.

Certain herbal supplements are also popular for promoting

lymphatic health. For example, burdock root is thought to contain natural diuretic characteristics that may help with the evacuation of excess fluid and toxins. Similarly, dandelion root is widely utilized for its potential to improve liver function and lymphatic drainage.

In response to these concerns, therapeutic approaches to lymphatic health have grown in favor, with a focus on natural therapies, dietary guidelines, and particular exercises to promote normal lymphatic function.

Exercise And Movement For Lymphatic Flow.

Physical exercise is essential for keeping a healthy lymphatic system. Unlike the circulatory system, the lymphatic system does not have a pump and instead relies on muscle contractions and body movement to adequately circulate lymph fluid. Including certain workouts and movement techniques may help to increase lymphatic flow.

Rebounding, or bouncing on a mini-trampoline, is a popular lymphatic support exercise. The up-and-down action increases gravity forces, which encourage lymphatic drainage. This low-impact workout is not only good for the lymphatic system but also easy on the joints, making it appropriate for people of all fitness levels.

Yoga is another kind of exercise that is often prescribed for lymphatic health. Certain yoga positions, including inversions and twists, are thought to promote lymphatic drainage by gently compressing and decompressing lymph nodes. Additionally, practicing deep diaphragmatic breathing during yoga helps improve general circulation, including lymphatic movement.

Regular cardiovascular activity, such as brisk walking, running, or swimming, may also help improve lymphatic function. Engaging in high-intensity exercises not only benefits cardiovascular health but also improves general circulation, allowing lymph to circulate more freely throughout the body.

Incorporating therapeutic methods into lymphatic health such as natural treatments, dietary recommendations, and exercise may be a proactive strategy to boost the immune system and general health. Individuals who include these methods in their everyday routines may enjoy increased lymphatic movement, less congestion, and better detoxification processes. It is critical to check with healthcare specialists before making large changes to one's diet, or exercise program, or applying new natural therapies, particularly for those who have pre-existing health concerns. Individuals may help to maintain a healthy lymphatic system by taking a comprehensive and proactive approach, which promotes maximum health and energy.

Hydration And Its Impact On Lymphatic Function

The human body is a complex and interrelated system, with each component playing an important part in general health. The lymphatic system is an often overlooked yet crucial feature. The lymphatic system is a network of tissues and organs that assist the body in eliminating toxins, waste, and other undesired substances. Proper hydration is essential for the lymphatic system's proper function.

The lymphatic system is based on the circulation of lymph, a colorless fluid containing white blood cells, throughout the body. This circulation is necessary for immune function because the lymphatic system filters and drains lymph, eliminating toxins and pathogens. Hydration is essential for maintaining lymph fluidity and promoting smooth flow throughout the body.

When the body is properly hydrated, the lymphatic system can effectively move immune cells and other important components, resulting in a stronger resistance against illnesses. Dehydration, on the other hand, may cause thicker lymphatic fluid, reducing its capacity to circulate freely. As a consequence, the immune response may be weakened, making the body more vulnerable to sickness.

In addition to boosting immune function, appropriate hydration helps to avoid lymphedema, a disease defined by the buildup of fluid in the tissues that often occurs when lymph nodes are removed during cancer treatment. Individuals who maintain appropriate hydration may reduce their chances of getting lymphedema and improve the overall health of their lymphatic system.

CHAPTER FOUR

External Therapies Include Massage And Manual Lymphatic Drainage

External treatments, such as massage and manual lymphatic drainage (MLD), are important in improving lymphatic system health and function. These treatments aim to increase lymphatic flow, reduce congestion, and improve the body's natural cleansing processes.

Massage For Lymphatic Support:

Massage, when given by a qualified practitioner, may benefit the lymphatic system. Gentle, rhythmic strokes focused at the lymph nodes promote lymphatic fluid flow, allowing waste and toxins to be removed more effectively. Massage also induces relaxation, which may assist in alleviating stress-related elements that lead to lymphatic system abnormalities.

Manual Lymphatic Drainage (Mld)

MLD is a specific massage method that stimulates the lymphatic system. MLD improves lymphatic fluid outflow from crowded regions by using gentle, precise motions. This therapy technique is very effective for those who have impaired lymphatic function, such as lymphedema. MLD may help reduce edema, improve circulation, and increase lymphatic system efficiency.

Massage and MLD both provide non-invasive, systemic lymphatic system assistance. Regular sessions may help to maintain healthy lymphatic function and avoid concerns with lymphatic congestion.

Herbal And Supplemental Support For The Lymphatic System

In addition to external therapy, herbal medicines, and supplements may help boost lymphatic system health. Certain herbs and supplements are known for their capacity to improve lymphatic function, decrease inflammation, and aid in detoxification.

Turmeric

Turmeric, recognized for its anti-inflammatory effects, has long been used to promote lymphatic function. Turmeric's primary ingredient, curcumin, has antioxidant and anti-inflammatory properties that may help reduce edema and promote lymphatic system health.

Echinacea

Echinacea is known for its immune-boosting qualities. This herb may help boost the immune response by assisting the lymphatic system in filtering and removing infections. During cold and flu season, echinacea pills are often used to boost the body's immune system.

Essential Fatty Acids

Fish oil and flaxseed oil include omega-3 fatty acids, which help to modulate inflammation and boost immunological function. Including these important fatty acids in your diet may help your lymphatic system function properly.

While herbal medicines and supplements may be beneficial, it is important to speak with a healthcare expert before adopting them into one's daily routine, particularly if one is using prescriptions or has pre-existing health concerns.

CHAPTER FIVE

Mind-Body Techniques For Holistic Wellness

Holistic health entails addressing the interdependence of mind and body. Incorporating mind-body techniques into everyday life may have a significant impact on the lymphatic system, encouraging balance and general health.

Meditation and deep breathing:

Mindfulness meditation and deep breathing techniques may assist in decreasing stress, which has been shown to influence lymphatic function. Stress management is essential for keeping a healthy lymphatic system since persistent stress may cause inflammation and decrease immune response.

Yoga

Yoga integrates physical postures, breathwork, and meditation, making it a complete practice that improves both the body and the mind.

Certain yoga positions, such as inversions and twists, are thought to aid lymphatic drainage by stimulating the flow of lymphatic fluid. Regular yoga practice may improve flexibility, relaxation, and general lymphatic health.

Hydrotherapy

Hydrotherapy refers to the use of water in different ways to improve health. Contrast hydrotherapy, or alternating hot and cold water in the shower, helps improve blood circulation and lymphatic movement. This simple technique may be readily adopted into a daily habit, helping to maintain the lymphatic system's general health.

Finally, lymphatic system health is important for general well-being, and many lifestyle choices may help it work optimally. Individuals may nurture their lymphatic health using a variety of strategies, including keeping hydrated, adding external treatments, herbal assistance, and mind-body activities. Individuals who take a holistic approach to well-being that addresses both the physical and emotional components may help to build a robust and efficient lymphatic system, laying the groundwork for a happier and more balanced existence.

Incorporating Essential Oils For Lymphatic Health

Essential oils, which are produced from plants and are recognized for their aromatic characteristics, have been used therapeutically in numerous civilizations for ages.

They have recently received attention for their ability to improve lymphatic health. The lymphatic system removes toxins, waste, and surplus fluids from the body, and essential oils are thought to help in this detoxification process.

Lemon essential oil, for example, is often regarded as excellent for lymphatic drainage. Its zesty scent is supposed to boost lymphatic movement and aid in toxin clearance. Similarly, grapefruit essential oil is said to have detoxifying effects, aiding the lymphatic system's cleaning processes. Another popular alternative is cypress essential oil, which has been shown to promote circulation and prevent fluid retention, thus adding to overall lymphatic health.

While essential oils may be used to help the lymphatic system, they must be used with care. Dilution and suitable application procedures are essential, and consultation with a competent aromatherapist or healthcare practitioner is recommended to ensure safe use.

Environmental Factors and Their Impact on the Lymphatic System

Environmental influences may either assist or inhibit the lymphatic system's activities, as they do with any other biological system. Sedentary lifestyles, poor dietary choices, exposure to environmental pollutants, and chronic stress are all factors that may harm the lymphatic system.

Lack of physical exercise, for example, may cause sluggish lymphatic flow, impeding the effective elimination of waste from the body. Processed meals rich in preservatives and chemicals may help to accumulate toxins, placing extra pressure on the lymphatic system. Environmental contaminants, such as pollution and pesticides, may also overburden the lymphatic system, impairing its capacity to operate properly.

Understanding these environmental influences enables people to make educated lifestyle decisions that benefit the health of their lymphatic system. Regular exercise, a balanced and nutrient-rich diet, appropriate hydration, and limiting exposure to environmental pollutants are all important factors in supporting lymphatic health.

CHAPTER SIX

Case Studies: Real-Life Examples Of Lymphatic Healing

Real-life experiences provide vital insights into the possible advantages of using essential oils to improve lymphatic function. Case studies emphasize unique experiences, offering information on the efficacy of natural lymphatic system assistance.

Sarah, a 45-year-old office worker, had recurrent swelling in her legs as a result of extended sitting at her desk. In search of a more holistic treatment, she began practicing daily self-massage using a diluted combination of cypress and grapefruit essential oils. Sarah experienced a considerable decrease in edema and pain after many weeks, which she attributed to the essential oils' lymphatic assistance.

Similarly, Mark, a 35-year-old fitness fanatic, struggled with post-workout muscular pain and occasional inflammation. He implemented a lymphatic massage program using diluted lemon essential oil, which provided relief from muscular soreness and enhanced recovery times.

These case studies highlight the individualized nature of essential oil use and its ability to supplement unique health journeys. However, it is important to understand that outcomes may vary, and individual factors such as allergies or pre-existing health concerns should be considered.

Preventive Strategies For Long-Term Lymphatic Health

In addition to using essential oils, taking preventative steps is critical to maintaining long-term lymphatic health. These strategies include lifestyle decisions and practices that promote the lymphatic system's normal function.

1. Hydration: Adequate water consumption is essential for proper lymphatic function. Staying hydrated helps to maintain the fluid balance required for effective lymphatic drainage.

2. Regular Exercise: Physical activity, especially rhythmic movements, promotes lymphatic circulation. Walking, swimming, and rebounding may all help to increase lymphatic flow.

3. A balanced diet that includes fruits, vegetables, and whole foods offers important nutrients for the

lymphatic system. Avoiding processed meals and limiting salt consumption may help improve lymphatic function.

4. Stress management: Prolonged stress might impede lymphatic function. Stress-relieving methods such as meditation, deep breathing, and yoga help improve general health, including the lymphatic system.

5. Body Brushing: Dry brushing the skin is said to stimulate the lymphatic system by increasing circulation and cleansing. This technique, when done carefully,

maybe a valuable complement to a self-care regimen.

Conclusion

To summarize, using essential oils for lymphatic health is a comprehensive strategy that works with the body's natural functions. Lemon, grapefruit, and cypress essential oils are regarded to be beneficial, although individual results may vary.

Environmental variables, such as lifestyle decisions and toxin exposure, have a substantial impact on lymphatic system performance. Real-life case studies demonstrate the potential advantages of using essential oils, highlighting the significance of tailored methods.

Individuals may maintain long-term lymphatic well-being by keeping hydrated, exercising regularly, eating a healthy diet, controlling stress, and adding body brushing into their daily routines.

Understanding and nourishing the lymphatic system may help people improve their overall health and energy, adopting a holistic approach to well-being.

www.ingramcontent.com/pod-product-compliance
Lightning Source LLC
Chambersburg PA
CBHW071127260726
48661CB00006B/2709